Bread Without Gluten:

Easy And Delicious Recipes

for a

Gluten-Free Lifestyle

DEDICATION

I would like to take a moment to thank my son, Paul and my friend Willis for their unwavering support and encouragement throughout the process of creating this cookbook. From taste-testing endless loaves of bread to providing feedback and constructive criticism, their love and support have been invaluable. This book would not be possible without without them and for that I say with all my heart, thank you and I love you both.

Bread Without Gluten:

Easy And Delicious Recipes for a Gluten-Free Lifestyle

TABLE OF CONTENTS

FOREWORD

I am thrilled to present to you this bread baking cookbook for those of you who are unable to tolerate gluten. As someone with a child that has struggled with gluten intolerance, I understand the frustration and disappointment that can come from not being able to enjoy some of life's simplest pleasures such as a warm bread, toast or any of the wheat products readily available..

But fear not--this cookbook is here to help you navigate the world of gluten-free bread baking with confidence and delicious results. Whether you are new to gluten-free cooking or a seasoned pro, this collection of recipes is sure to inspire and excite your taste buds.

One of the biggest challenges when it comes to gluten-free baking is achieving the right texture and flavor in bread. Gluten is a unique protein found in wheat, barley, and rye that gives bread its structure and elasticity. When baking without gluten, it can be difficult to mimic this same texture and rise, leading to dense, crumbly loaves that lack the signature chewiness of traditional bread.

That's why each recipe in this cookbook has been carefully crafted and tested to ensure that you not only get a great-tasting loaf of bread but also one that has the perfect texture and crumb. From light and airy sandwich bread to hearty, rustic loaves, there is something here for everyone, regardless of your level of baking expertise.

So, I invite you to grab your apron, preheat your oven, and dive into the wonderful world of gluten-free bread baking with this cookbook as your guide. May these recipes bring joy, comfort, and deliciousness to your table, and may each loaf you bake be a testament to the power of perseverance and creativity in the face of dietary restrictions.

Happy baking!

Warmly,
Pansy Worthy

INTRODUCTION

Welcome to "Bread Without Gluten: Easy And Delicious Recipes for a Gluten-Free Lifestyle"! I am a Mom, and I am thrilled to share with you my passion for baking gluten free breads. As a busy single mom with a son on the autism spectrum and not having the time to prepare fresh bread, I was just buying supermarket bread and gluten products for my family. However, when my son was diagnosed with a digestive disorder and doctors had given up on him, saying that it was all in his head and no help was available, every day for my son was a day closer to death a few years ago.

I radically changed our whole way of eating. I had to completely change the way I approached baking. Suddenly, all of our favorite bread recipes were off-limits, and I was faced with the challenge of finding ways to create delicious gluten-free alternatives.

After countless hours in the kitchen experimenting with different flours, ingredients, and techniques, I am proud to say that I have developed a collection of gluten-free bread recipes that are not only tasty and satisfying but also easy to make at home. In this cookbook, I have compiled some of our family's favorite recipes, Whether you are new to the world of gluten-free baking or have been living a gluten-free lifestyle for years, I hope that this cookbook will inspire you to get creative in the kitchen and enjoy delicious bread once again. There is something for everyone in these pages.

I know that navigating the world of gluten-free baking can be overwhelming at first, but I want to assure you that with a little practice and patience, you can create bread that is just as delicious and satisfying as its gluten-filled counterparts. Whether you are baking for yourself, a family member, or a friend with gluten intolerance, I hope that these recipes will bring joy and comfort to your kitchen.

Finally, I want to thank you, the reader, for choosing to explore the world of gluten-free baking with me. I hope that the recipes in this cookbook bring a little more joy and deliciousness to your gluten-free lifestyle.

With Love,
Pansy Worthy

Bread Without Gluten:

Easy And Delicious Recipes

for a

Gluten-Free Lifestyle

Quinoa Millet Bread

Dry Ingredients

2/3 cup quinoa flour

2/3 cup millet flour

3/4 cup brown rice flour

1/4 cup ground flax seed

2 tablespoons almond flour

2 teaspoons unflavored gelatin

1/2 teaspoon salt

1 tablespoon baking soda

Wet Ingredients

1 1/4 cup milk

1 tablespoon honey

3 eggs

3 tablespoon plain yogurt

1 1/2 tablespoons melted coconut oil

1 teaspoon apple cider vinegar

Instruction:

Grease and line with parchment paper 9x5 inch bread and set aside. Preheat oven to 350F/180C. Put all dry ingredient into a bowl and mix thoroughly. Whisk all the wet ingredient-eggs, milk, honey, yogurt, coconut oil, and apple cider vinegar in another bowl. Add egg mixture to dry ingredient and stir well to combine thoroughly. Pour the mixture into the prepared bread pan.

Bake for 30 minutes or until bake. Use a knife or toothpick to test if bread is baked by sticking the knife or toothpick in the middle of the bread. If the knife or toothpick comes out clean, then bread is done. Allow the bread to cool before cutting. Store in fridge for up to five days, or slice and freeze for up to three months.

Banana Oat Bread

Ingredients

3 large ripe bananas (speckled bananas)

2 large eggs

1/4 cup pure maple syrup (or honey)

1/2 teaspoon baking soda

1/4 teaspoon sea salt

1/2 teaspoon apple cider vinegar

2 cups old fashioned rolled oats

1/4 cup coconut oil or olive oil

Instruction:

Preheat oven to 350°F/180C. Grease and line loaf pan with parchment paper and set aside. Crack the eggs into a bowl. Add the olive oil, honey, apple cider vinegar and whisk until ingredients are well combined. Mashed the ripe bananas in a separate bowl. Add mash ripe bananas to the mixture. Put rolled oats in a blender and blender into flour. Add the oats, sea salt and baking soda to the liquid mixture. Stir until well combined. Pour batter into greased loaf pan. Bake for 30-35 minutes or until bake. To test if cake is bake, insert a toothpick in the center and if the toothpick comes out clean, then it is bake.

Allow bread loaf to cool before cutting. Store bread in fridge for up to a week or sliced and stored in freezer for up to 3 months

Seed Bread- Flour-less Bread

Dry Ingredients:

3 ounce of sesame seeds

3 ounce of sunflower seeds

3 ounce of walnuts, chopped

3 ounce of pumpkin seeds

3 ounce of flax seed

3 ounce of chia seed

½ teaspoon of baking soda

1/2 teaspoon sea salt

Wet Ingredients

4 egg white

1/2 teaspoon apple cider vinegar

3 1/2 ounce of water

Instruction:

Preheat oven to 350 F/180C. Grease and line loaf pan with parchment paper. Set loaf pan aside. Crack the eggs and separate egg white from the yellow. Whisk egg whites with sea salt. In this recipe we will be using the egg whites only. Egg yellow can be stored in the refrigerator and use in other meals. Add water, apple cider vinegar and baking soda to the whisk eggs. Put all the seeds in a blender and grind into fine flour or your desire texture. You can choose to grind some and chop some so that you bread can have seed in it. Add the seed flour to the mixture and mix well. Add walnut and give a good stir. Pour mixture into the greased loaf pan. Even out the top with a spatula.

 Bake bread for 50 minutes or until bake. Allow to cool before cutting. Bread can be stored in fridge for one week or sliced and freeze for up to 3 months in freezer.

Brown Rice Oats Bread

Dry Ingredients

2 cups brown rice flour

1 1/2 cup of gluten free oats

3 tablespoon flax seed

1/2 tsp sea salt

1/2 tsp baking soda

Wet Ingredients

I tsp apple cider vinegar

1/8 cup of raw honey

1/4 cup coconut oil

1 1/2 cup whole organic milk

3 eggs

Instruction:

Grease loaf pan and line with parchment paper and set aside. Parchment paper is optional. It makes the loaf easier to remove from the loaf pan. Whisk eggs. Add all the other wet ingredient apple cider vinegar, raw honey, coconut oil, and milk. Stir vigorously until well combined. Grind gluten free oats, flax seed and into flour. Add all dry ingredients (brown rice flour, oats flour and flax flour, salt, baking soda) and stir until well combined. The mixture should be thicken. If too runny, add some more brown rice flour. If too thick, add more milk.

Transfer mixture to the grease loaf pan and smooth top out as best you can with a spatula. Bake at 350F/180C for about 20-30 minutes or until top turns slight brown. Stick a knife or toothpick in the middle of the bread and when the knife or toothpick comes out smooth the bread is done. Wait until the bread is cool, then remove from the pan and slice.

This bread will not last long as it is very delicious. You can slice the bread and store in fridge for about a week or slice and freeze for about 3 months.

Millet Bread

Ingredient

2 1/2 cup of millet flour

1/2 tsp of baking soda

3 tbsp plain yogurt

3 organic eggs

3 tbsp raw honey

1tsp lemon juice or apple cider vinegar

1/2 Tsp sea salt or pink Himalayan salt

1 cup organic whole milk

1 pack unflavored gelatin

Grease bread pan and line with parchment paper. Set bread pan aside. Preheat oven at 350F/180C. In a large bowl mix the dry ingredients, millet flour, baking soda, sea salt and unflavored gelatin. Whisked eggs and add all the wet ingredients- lemon juice or apple cider vinegar, raw honey, organic whole milk, and yogurt. Add the dry ingredients you combined in the bowl. Stir until well combined. Using clean and moist hand form a ball. Shape the dough into a loaf shape as best as you can.

Placed the dough into the grease loaf pan and bake for about 40 minutes until slightly golden brown. Use a toothpick to test if bread is done. Insert toothpick in the middle of the bread and pull it out. If the toothpick comes out clean, then the bread is done.

Allow the bread to cool before removing from the pan and slice. You can slice the bread and store in fridge for about a week or slice and freeze for about 3 months.

Almond Flour Bread

Ingredients

2 cups blanched almond flour

1/2 teaspoon baking soda

1/4 teaspoon sea salt

3 tablespoons freshly ground flax seed

4 large eggs

1 teaspoon fresh lemon juice

1 tablespoon honey or agave

1/2 cup butter melted or melted coconut butter

1/2 cup milk of your choice

Instruction

Preheat oven to 180C/350F. Grease and line a bread pan or loaf pan with parchment paper. In a bowl, add all dry ingredient-almond flour, sea salt, baking soda and freshly ground flax seed and mix well. In a larger bowl, crack open the eggs and pour into bowl. Whisk the eggs. Add melted butter, milk, honey and lemon juice to the eggs and whisk until well combined. Stir in the dry ingredient and stir well until evenly distributed.   Pour batter into loaf pan and even out with a spatula.

Bake for 30 minutes or until toothpick comes clean. Let the bread cool before slicing. Bread can be stored in the refrigerator for up to 5 days or sliced an stored in the freezer for about 6 months. Enjoy.

Flour-less Peanut Butter Bread

Ingredient

1 cup peanut butter

4 eggs

2 cups oat flour

1/2 tsp baking soda

1/2 teaspoon sea salt

1/4 cup honey

1 tsp apple cider vinegar

Instruction

Preheat the oven to 300F. Grease and line the loaf pan and set aside. Cracked open eggs into a bowl and whisk eggs. Add the apple cider vinegar, honey, sea salt, baking soda, peanut butter and oat flour. Mix all until evenly distributed. Pour mixture into the grease loaf pan and bake for 25 minutes or until golden brown. Allow to cool before slicing. Enjoy and keep in the fridge for up to a week.

Chocolate Zucchini Bread

Ingredients:

Dry ingredients:

Almond flour, 1 ½ cups

Flax meal flour, ¼ cup

Coconut flour, ¼ cup

Cacao powder, ½ cup

Baking soda, 2 tsp

Cinnamon powder, 1 tsp

 Kosher salt, ½ tsp

Instant coffee, 1tsp

Chocolate chips, 1 cup, unsweetened

Wet ingredients:

 Eggs, 3 large

Applesauce, ¼ cup

Maple syrup, ½ cup

Yogurt, 3 tbsp

Coconut oil, ½ cup

Vanilla extract, 2 tsp

Apple cider vinegar, 1 tbsp

Zucchini, 1 ½ cups, grated

Instructions:

Preheat the oven to 350 degrees Fahrenheit. Add all dry ingredients to the mixing bowl and stir to combine. Add wet ingredients (except zucchini) to another mixing bowl. Stir well. Add zucchini to the wet ingredient and stir thoroughly. Pour the dry ingredients into the wet ingredients and stir to evenly distribute ingredients. Add chocolate chips and fold in. Pour the batter into a greased loaf pan lined with parchment paper. Sprinkle the top with remaining chocolate chips. Bake for 1 hour. Serve!

Pumpkin Bread

Ingredients:

Pumpkin puree, 1 cup

Eggs, 3

Coconut oil, ¼ cup

Vanilla extract, 1 tsp

Almond flour, 1 cup

Flax meal flour, ½ cup

Apple cider vinegar, 1 tbsp

Agave, 3 tbsp

Yogurt, 3 tbsp

Baking soda, 1¼ tsp

Pumpkin pie spice, 2 tsp

Cinnamon, 1 tsp

Ground ginger, ½ tsp

Sea salt, ½ tsp

Pumpkin seeds, 2 tbsp, shelled

Instructions:

Preheat the oven to 350 degrees Fahrenheit. Add vanilla, coconut oil, apple cider vinegar, agave, yogurt, eggs, and pumpkin to a bowl. Using an electric mixer to combine well. Add salt, ginger, cinnamon, pumpkin pie spice, baking soda, almond flour, and flax meal flour to the bowl and combine. Line a greased loaf pan with parchment paper. Transfer the batter to the loaf pan and sprinkle with pumpkin seeds. Bake for 35 minutes. Serve!

Potato Bread

Ingredients:

Potato, ¾ lb

Whole milk, 2 cups

Agave, 1 tbsp

Active dry yeast, 4 ½ tsp

Butter, ¼ cup, melted

Sea salt, 1 tbsp

Gluten-free flour, 7 to 8 cups

Instructions:

Peel potatoes and cut them into chunks. Place a saucepan with water on the stove and bring to a boil. Add the potato and lower the heat and cook until tender. Allow it to cool and drain it. Mash potato with a fork and set aside. Now, add milk to a saucepan and warm it. Add agave to the milk and combine well. Add yeast to the milk mixture and stir.

Set aside and allow the milk mixture to stand for 10 minutes. After 10 minutes add gluten free flour, sea salt, melted butter, milk, and mashed potatoes, to the yeast mixture and combine well. Allow it to knead in the mixer on low until smooth for 5 to 7 minutes or using your hands to knead for 2 to 3 minutes. Transfer the dough to a greased bowl and cover it with a clean kitchen towel. Allow it to rise for 1 hour.

Divide the dough in half and transfer each half into greased loaf pan. Allow it to rise for an additional 45 minutes. Preheat the oven to 350 degrees Fahrenheit. Bake for 45 to 55 minutes until golden brown. Serve!

White Bread

Ingredients:

Active dry yeast, 2 ¼ tsp

Warm water, ¼ cup

Agave, 1 tbsp

Milk, 2 cups

Sea salt, 2 tsp

Butter, 2 tbsp, melted

Gluten-free flour, 6 cups

Instructions:

Add yeast, and warm water to a bowl and combine well. Set aside for 10 minutes Add butter, agave, and milk to another bowl and combine well. Add flour and sea salt to the milk mixture. Stir well. Add yeast mixture and combine well. Place the dough onto the floured surface and knead until smooth. Place the dough into the grease bowl and cover it with plastic wrap. Allow it to rise for 1 hour.

Place the dough onto the cutting board. Roll the dough into a log. Place the log dough into the greased loaf pan. Allow it to rise for an additional 30 to 40 minutes. Preheat the oven to 400 degrees Fahrenheit. Bake for 25 to 30 minutes.

Serve and enjoy!

Brown Rice Focaccia Bread

Ingredients:

Brown Rice flour, 2 ¼ cups

Dry yeast, 2 tsp

Sea salt, ¾ tsp

Baking powder, 1 tsp

Milk, ¾ cup plus 2 tbsp

Eggs, 2

Yogurt, 3 tablespoon

Extra virgin olive oil,¼ cups

Extra virgin olive oil, 2 tbsp, for coating

Instructions:

Add all dry ingredients to the mixing bowl and whisk to combine. Add almond milk into a pot and warm. Add yeast and olive oil to the almond milk and allow it to stand for 5 minutes to cool down. After 5 minutes, add eggs and yogurt to the liquid mixture and combine well. Add the dry ingredients to the wet ingredients and combine well.

Cover the dough with plastic wrap and set aside for 1 hour. Dough should double in size. Place the dough on a parchment paper-lined baking tray. With greased hands, spread the dough out. Make indentation in the dough using your fingers. Dust with brown rice flour. Preheat the oven to 375 degrees Fahrenheit. Add extra olive oil to a dish and brush it over the dough. Bake for 20 to 25 minutes until golden and crusty. Serve!

Sun-Dried Tomato Olive Bread

Ingredients:

Olives, ½ cup, chopped

Sun-dried tomatoes, ½ cup, chopped

Brown Rice flour, 2 cups

Baking soda, 1 tsp

Lemon zest, 1 tsp

Oregano, ½ tsp

Basil, ½ tsp

Pink or Sea Salt, ½ tsp

Eggs, 3

Greek yogurt, 1/3 cup

Honey, 3 tbsp

Lemon juice, 1 tbsp

Milk, 1 ¼ tbsp

Olive oil, 2 ½ tbsp

Instructions:

Preheat the oven to 340 degrees Fahrenheit. Grease the loaf pan lined with parchment paper. Add chopped tomatoes and chopped olives to a bowl and combine. Set it aside. Add pink or sea salt, basil, oregano, lemon zest, baking soda, and brown rice flour to another bowl and whisk to combine. Add olive oil, milk, eggs, lemon juice and yogurt in a medium bowl and combine with an electric mixer on medium speed until smooth. Add the flour mixture with the wet mixture and combine well. Then, fold in the chopped tomato and olive in the mixture.

Transfer it to the greased loaf pan. Bake for 40 minutes. Serve!

Peaches and Cream Bread

Ingredients:

Peach filling:

Peaches, 2, thinly sliced

Lemon juice, ½ tbsp

Agave, 2 tbsp

Gelatin, unflavored, 1 pack

Sweet dough bread:

Milk, warm, ½ cup plus ½ tbsp

Active dry yeast, 1 ¾ tsp

Rice flour, 2 ½ cups

Salt, ¼ tsp

Agave, 2 ½ tbsp

Egg, 1

Butter, 2 tbsp, softened

Cream cheese frosting:

2 tbsp vanilla extract

2 tbsp melted butter

2 tbsp agave,

4 oz cream cheese,

1 tbsp cinnamon powder

Instruction

Add lemon juice and peaches to the bowl and toss to combine. Add gelatin and agave to the bowl and combine well. Set it aside.

Sweet dough bread:

Add yeast and 1/2 cup of warm milk to the small bowl and combine well. Allow it to stand for 10 minutes. Add the salt and rice flour to another mixing bowl and combine well. Add vanilla, butter, egg and agave and stir well. Add milk and yeast mixture to the flour mixture and combine well. Place the dough on the floured surface and roll it into a ball. Wrap it in plastic wrap and place it in the fridge for an 2 hours to allow it to rise.

Place the dough on the floured surface and knead it to form a loaf. Grease and flour the loaf pan. Place the dough in the loaf pan and rest it for an additional 40 minutes. Preheat the oven to 350 degrees Fahrenheit. Brush the dough with remaining 1/2 tbsp of milk. Bake for 45 to 50 minutes. Slice bread when cool.

Prepare the cream cheese frosting: Add vanilla, agave, cream cheese, cinnamon powder and butter to a bowl and combine well. Frost slice of bread with cream cheese frosting and topped with peach fillings. Serve and enjoy.

Oat Banana Raisin Nut Bread

Ingredients:

Oatmeal flour, 2 cups,

Coconut flour, 4 tbsp

Raisins, 1 cup

Agave, ¾ cups

Ground cinnamon, ½ tsp

Sea salt, ¼ tsp

Apple cider vinegar, 1 tbsp

Vanilla extract, 1 tsp

Baking soda, 1 tsp

Eggs, 3

Banana 3, ripe and mashed

Butter, 4 tbsp, melted

Walnuts, ¼ cup, chopped

Instructions:

Preheat the oven to 350 degrees Fahrenheit. Add baking soda, sea salt, ground cinnamon raisins, oatmeal flour, and coconut flour to the bowl and combine well. Add eggs, agave, mashed banana, apple cider vinegar, melted butter, and vanilla extract to another bowl. Mix well. Pour wet ingredients into the dry ingredients and combine well. Pour the batter to loaf pan. Top with walnuts. Bake for 40 to 50 minutes until bake. Allow to cool before slicing. Serve!

Almond Flour Bread

Ingredients:

Eggs, 5

Coconut oil, 5 tbsp

Apple cider vinegar, 1 tsp

Kosher salt, ¼ tsp

Almond flour, 1 ¾ cup, blanched

Baking soda, ¾ tsp

Instructions:

Preheat the oven to 350 degrees Fahrenheit. Grease and line the loaf pan with parchment paper. In a bowl crack and whisk eggs. Add coconut oil and apple cider vinegar and whisk. Add almond flour, salt and baking soda to the bowl and whisk to combine evenly. Pour the batter to the loaf pan. Bake for 30 to 40 minutes. Serve!

Millet Raisin Bread

Ingredients:

Active dry yeast, 2 tsp

Agave, 1 tsp

Water, 1 cup, warm

Millet flour, 1 cup

Raisin, 1 cup

Gelatin, unflavored, 1 pack

Brown rice flour, ½ cup

Flax meal, ¼ cup

Salt, 1 tsp

Eggs, 2

Olive oil, 3 tbsp

Yogurt, 3 tbsp

Instructions:

Add warm water, agave, and yeast to the bowl and combine well. Allow it to get frosty for 10 to 15 minutes. Add salt, flax meal, brown rice flour, gelatin, and millet flour to another bowl mix and set aside. In a another bowl, add olive oil, yogurt and eggs and whisk to combine well. Then, add the yeast mixture and stir well. Add all the dry ingredients and combine well. Transfer the dough a greased lined loaf pan. Cover with damp wet paper towel. Allow it to rise for 45 to 90 minutes. Preheat the oven to 350 degrees Fahrenheit. When the dough has risen, bake for 40 to 45 minutes. Serve!

Brown Rice Bread

Ingredients:

Brown rice flour, 2 cups

Milk, 1 ½ cups, warm

Greek Yogurt, 3 tbsp

Coconut oil, ¼ cup

Agave, 2 tbsp

Gelatin, unflavored, 1 pack

Egg whites, 2

Baking soda, 1 tsp, sifted

Lemon Juice 1 tbsp

Sea salt, ½ tsp

Instructions:

Preheat the oven to 350 degrees Fahrenheit. Add sea salt, baking soda, gelatin, and brown rice flour to the mixing bowl and combine well. Set aside. Add egg whites, agave, lemon juice, coconut oil, yogurt and milk to a bowl and combine well. Add dry ingredients to the wet ingredients and combine well. Pour the mixture into a greased lined loaf pan.

Bake for 1 hour until golden brown. Insert toothpick into the middle of the bread to test if done. If not, return to oven for a few more minutes and repeat the test. Allow to cool before cutting. Serve and enjoy!

Oatmeal Bread

Ingredients:

Almond milk, 2 ½ cups

Butter, 4 tbsp, softened

Agave, ½ cup

Apple cider vinegar, 1½ tbsp

Baking soda, 1½ tsp

Sea salt, 1 ½ tsp

Oatmeal flour, 2 ½ cup

Flax meal flour, 2 tbsp

Rolled oats, 1 cup

Eggs, 2

Egg yolk , 1, mixed with water to make egg wash

Instructions:

Add butter and eggs to a bowl and whisked. Add agave, apple cider vinegar and almond milk to the eggs mixture and stir well. Add baking soda, sea salt, flax meal flour and oatmeal flour and combine well Add the roll oats and fold in. Transfer the dough to the greased lined bread pan Bake for 30 minutes.

Remove and brush with egg wash. Bake for an additional 10 minutes. Test with a toothpick or knife by inserting it in the middle of the loaf. If it comes out clean, bread is bake. If not done, bake for a few more minutes. Serve!

Seed and Nut Bread

Ingredients:

Rolled oats, 1 ½ cups

Pumpkin seeds, chopped ½ cup

Sunflower seeds, chopped ½ cup

Hazelnuts, chopped ½ cup

Almonds, chopped ¼ cup

Sesame seeds, chopped 1/3 cup

Ground flaxseed meal, ¼ cup

Chia seeds, chopped 2 tbsp

Psyllium husk, 3 tbsp

Sea Salt, 1 ½ tsp

Agave, 2 tbsp

Coconut oil, 3 tbsp

Milk, 1 ½ cups

Instructions:

Preheat the oven to 375 degrees Fahrenheit. Add all dry ingredients to the bowl and combine well. Add milk, coconut oil, and agave the bowl and whisk to combine. Add dry ingredients to the wet ingredients and stir well. Transfer the mixture to the greased lined loaf pan. Bake for 45 minutes. Allow to cool before serving. Serve!

Quinoa Bread

Ingredients:

Quinoa, 2 cups, cooked

Oat flour, 1 cup

Yogurt, plain, 3 tbsp

Baking soda, 1 ½ tsp

Apple cider vinegar, 1 ½ tbsp

Salt, ¼ tsp

Coconut oil, 3 tbsp

Almond milk, 2 cups

Agave, 1 tbsp

Instructions:

Preheat the oven to 400 degrees Fahrenheit. Grease the loaf pan with coconut oil and lined with parchment paper. Add quinoa to the food processor and pulse until smooth. Transfer the mixture to the bowl. Add vinegar, agave, and almond milk to the bowl and stir well. Add coconut oil and yogurt and stir well. Add sea salt, baking soda, and oat flour and combine well. Transfer it to the greased loaf pan. Sprinkle with sesame seeds. Bake for 1 hour. Serve!

Cinnamon Bread

Ingredients:

Dry ingredients:

Almond flour, 2 ½ cups

Baking soda, 1 tsp

Gelatin, unflavored, 1 pack

Wet ingredients:

Eggs, 3

Coconut oil, ½ cup

Yogurt, 1 1/3 cups

Apple cider vinegar, 1 tbsp

Vanilla extract, 2 tsp

Agave, 1 cup

Cinnamon sweetener:

Unsalted butter, 4 tbsp, melted

Cinnamon powder, 1 ½ tbsp

Agave, ¾ cup

Instructions:

Preheat the oven to 350 degrees Fahrenheit. Grease the loaf pan and line with baking paper. Add dry ingredients to a bowl and combine well. Add wet ingredients in another bowl and combine well. Add cinnamon sweetener ingredients in a small bowl and mix well. Set aside. Add dry ingredients to wet ingredients and combine well. Pour half the mixture into the loaf pan. Pour half the cinnamon sweetener in the loaf pan. Pour remaining batter. Bake for 12 to 15 minutes.

Remove from oven and add the remaining cinnamon mixture over it. Bake for 40 minutes or until brown. Test if baked using a toothpick or knife. Serve!

Oatmeal Raisin Bread

Ingredients:

Old-fashioned rolled oats, Gluten free, 1 cup   Oatmeal flour, gluten free, 1 ½ cups

Raisins, 1 cup, chopped

Baking soda, 1 tbsp

Sea salt, 1 tsp

Cinnamon powder, 1 tsp

Nutmeg, 1 tsp

Orange zest, ½ tsp

Orange juice, ½ cup

Yogurt, 3 tbsp

Butter, 2 tbsp, melted

Agave, ½ cup

Eggs, 3

Almond Milk, ¼ cup

Instructions:

In a bowl, add all the dry ingredients except the raisins and stir to distribute evenly. Set aside. In a larger bowl, crack and whisk the eggs. Add melted butter, orange juice, agave, milk and orange zest and whisk to combine. Add all the dry ingredients and raisins and mix well. Grease and floured the bread pan. Bake in the preheated oven at 350 degrees Fahrenheit for 45 minutes until golden brown or until bake. Serve warm or allow to cool fully and store for later.

Keto Bread

Ingredients:

Eggs, 6

Butter, ½ cup, melted

Coconut oil, 2 tbsp

Agave, 2 tbsp

Almond flour, 2 cups

Baking soda, 1 tsp

Lemon juice, 1 tbsp

Flax meal, 2 tbsp

Sea salt, ½ tsp

Instructions:

Preheat the oven to 350 degrees Fahrenheit. Add eggs to the bowl and beat on high speed using a mixer for 1 to 2 minutes. Add coconut oil, melted butter, lemon juice, agave and mix. Then, add sea salt, baking soda, flax meal and almond flour and combine well. Pour the batter in a oiled loaf pan lined with baking paper. Bake for 45 minutes. Cut it into slices when cool. Serve or store until later.

Keto Sandwich Bread

Ingredients:

Almond flour, 2 cups, blanched

Baking soda, 1 tsp

Lemon juice, 1 tbsp

Salt, ½ tsp

Eggs, 4

Ground flax seed, 3 tbsp

Unsalted butter, ½ cup, melted

Almond milk, ½ cup

Agave, ½ tbsp

Sesame seeds, 1 tbsp

Instructions:

Preheat the oven to 350 degrees Fahrenheit. Grease the loaf pan and line it with parchment paper. Add baking soda and lemon juice to a bowl and combine well. Add eggs to the bowl and beat with a hand mixer on medium speed for 3 to 5 minutes. Add agave, almond milk, butter, and combine well. Add all the other dry ingredients and combine well. Transfer the batter to the greased loaf pan and bake for 40 to 45 minutes. Enjoy!

Classic Oatmeal Bread

Ingredients:

2 1/4 cups warm water

1 tablespoon active dry yeast

1/4 cup honey

2 tablespoons vegetable oil

2 teaspoons salt

3 cups gluten free flour

2 cups rolled oats

Instructions:

In a large bowl, combine warm water, yeast, and honey. Let sit for 5 minutes until foamy.Stir in vegetable oil, honey and salt. Gradually add gluten free flour and rolled oats, mixing until a dough forms. Knead the dough on a floured surface for 5-7 minutes, until smooth and elastic. Place the dough in a greased bowl, cover with a towel, and let rise in a warm place for 1 hour. Punch down the dough and shape into a loaf. Place in a greased loaf pan. Let rise for another 30 minutes. Preheat oven to 350°F (180°C). Bake bread for 30-35 minutes, until golden brown and bake. Allow to cool before slicing and serving.

Cinnamon Swirl Oatmeal Bread

Ingredients:

1 package instant oatmeal, any flavor

1/4 cup warm water

1 tablespoon active dry yeast

1/4 cup honey

2 tablespoons vegetable oil

2 teaspoons sea salt

3 cups bread flour

2 teaspoons cinnamon

1/4 cup brown sugar

Instructions:

In a small bowl, mix the active dry yeast with warm water and let sit for 5 minutes. In a large bowl, combine honey, vegetable oil, sea salt and oatmeal with the mixture. Gradually add bread flour and knead until a dough forms. Let rise for 1 hour in a warm place. In a small bowl, mix cinnamon and brown sugar. Roll out the dough into a rectangle and sprinkle the cinnamon sugar mixture. Roll up the dough and place in a greased loaf pan. Let rise for another 30 minutes. Bake at 350°F (180°C) for 30-35 minutes. Cool before slicing and serving.

Cranberry Oatmeal Bread

Ingredients:

1 1/2 cups warm water

1 tablespoon active dry yeast

1/4 cup honey

2 tablespoons olive oil

2 teaspoons salt

3 cups gluten free flour

1 cup rolled oats

1 cup dried cranberries

Instructions:

In a large bowl, combine warm water, yeast, and honey. Let sit for 5 minutes. Stir in olive oil and salt. Gradually add gluten free flour, rolled oats, and dried cranberries. Knead the dough for 5-7 minutes until smooth and elastic. Place the dough in a greased bowl, cover with a towel, and let rise for 1 hour. Shape the dough into a loaf and place in a greased pan. Let rise for 30 minutes.. Preheat oven to 350°F (180°C). Bake for 30-35 minutes until golden brown. Cool, slice, and serve.

Pumpkin Oatmeal Bread

Ingredients:

1 1/2 cups warm water

1 tablespoon active dry yeast

1/4 cup honey

2 tablespoons coconut oil

2 teaspoons salt

3 cups gluten free flour

1 cup rolled oats

1 cup canned pumpkin puree

1 teaspoon pumpkin pie spice

Instructions:

In a large bowl, combine warm water, yeast, and honey. Let sit for 5 minutes until foamy.. Stir in coconut oil and salt. Gradually add gluten free flour, rolled oats, pumpkin puree, and pumpkin pie spice. Knead the dough for 5-7 minutes until smooth and elastic. Place the dough in a greased bowl, cover with a towel, and let rise for 1 hour. Shape the dough into a loaf and place in a greased pan. Let rise for 30 minutes. Preheat oven to 350°F (180°C). Bake for 30-35 minutes until golden brown. Cool, slice, and serve.

Maple Oatmeal Bread

Ingredients:

1 1/2 cups warm water

1 tablespoon active dry yeast

1/4 cup maple syrup

2 tablespoons coconut oil

2 teaspoons sea salt

3 cups gluten free bread flour

1 cup rolled oats

Instructions:

In a large bowl, combine warm water, yeast, and maple syrup. Let sit for 5 minutes until foamy. Stir in coconut oil and sea salt. Gradually add gluten free bread flour and rolled oats, mixing until a dough forms. Knead the dough on a floured surface for 5-7 minutes, until smooth and elastic. Place the dough in a greased bowl, cover with a towel, and let rise in a warm place for 1 hour. Punch down the dough and shape into a loaf. Place in a greased loaf pan. Let rise for another 30 minutes. Preheat oven to 350°F (180°C). Bake bread for 30-35 minutes, until golden brown and baked. Allow to cool before slicing and serving.

Coconut Flour Bread

Ingredients:

1 cup coconut flour

3 eggs

1/4 cup melted coconut oil

3 tbsp plain yogurt

1 tbsp agave

1/2 tsp baking powder

1/2 tsp sea salt

Instructions:

Preheat oven to 350°F and grease a loaf pan. In a mixing bowl, whisk together coconut flour, baking powder, and sea salt. Add in eggs, yogurt, agave and melted coconut oil, stirring until well combined. Pour batter into loaf pan and smooth out the top. Bake for 30-35 minutes or until a toothpick inserted in the center comes out clean. Let cool before slicing and serving.

Paleo Coconut Flour Bread

Ingredients:

1 cup coconut flour

4 eggs

1/4 cup coconut oil, melted

3 tbsp Greek yogurt

1/2 tsp baking soda

1/2 tsp sea salt

Instructions:

Preheat oven to 350°F and grease a loaf pan. In a mixing bowl, combine coconut flour, baking soda, and sea salt. Add in eggs. Yogurt, melted coconut oil, mixing until smooth. Pour batter into loaf pan and bake for 40-45 minutes or until a toothpick inserted in the center comes out clean. Let cool before slicing and serving.

Coconut Flour Zucchini Bread

Ingredients:

1 cup coconut flour

3 tablespoon plain yogurt

4 eggs

1/4 cup honey

1/4 cup coconut oil, melted

1 tsp cinnamon

1 tsp baking powder

1 cup shredded zucchini

1/4 tsp sea salt

Instructions:

Preheat oven to 350°F and grease a loaf pan. In a mixing bowl, whisk together coconut flour, cinnamon, sea salt and baking powder. Add in eggs, honey, yogurt and melted coconut oil, stirring until well combined. Fold in shredded zucchini until evenly distributed. Pour batter into loaf pan and bake for 45-50 minutes or until a toothpick inserted in the center comes out clean. Let cool before slicing and serving.

Coconut Flour Banana Bread

Ingredients:

1 1/2 cups coconut flour

4 ripe bananas, mashed

4 eggs

3 tbsp plain yogurt

1/3 cup coconut oil, melted

1 tsp vanilla extract

1 tsp cinnamon

1 tsp baking powder

1/4 tsp sea salt

Instructions:

Preheat oven to 350°F and grease a loaf pan.

In a mixing bowl, combine coconut flour, cinnamon, sea salt and baking powder. Add in mashed bananas, eggs, melted coconut oil, yogurt and vanilla extract, mixing until smooth. Pour batter into loaf pan and bake for 50-55 minutes or until a toothpick inserted in the center comes out clean. Let cool before slicing and serving.

Coconut Flour Lemon Poppy Seed Bread

Ingredients:

1 cup coconut flour

4 eggs

1/4 cup honey

3 tablespoon yogurt

1/4 cup coconut oil, melted

Zest of 1 lemon

Juice of 1 lemon

1/2 tsp baking soda

1/4 tsp sea salt

2 tbsp poppy seeds

Instructions:

Preheat oven to 350°F and grease a loaf pan. In a mixing bowl, whisk together coconut flour, lemon zest, sea salt and baking soda. Add in eggs, honey, yogurt, melted coconut oil, lemon juice, and poppy seeds, stirring until well combined. Pour batter into loaf pan and bake for 40-45 minutes or until a toothpick inserted in the center comes out clean. Let cool before slicing and serving.

Sprouted Gluten-Free Quinoa Bread

Ingredients:

1 cup quinoa flour

1/2 cup sprouted quinoa seeds

1/4 cup flaxseed meal

1/4 cup coconut flour

3 tbsp plain yogurt

1 tsp baking powder

1/2 tsp sea salt

2 eggs

1/4 cup almond milk

2 tbsp honey

Instructions:

Preheat your oven to 350°F and grease a loaf pan. In a large mixing bowl, combine quinoa flour, sprouted quinoa seeds, flaxseed meal, coconut flour, baking powder, and sea salt. In a separate bowl, whisk together eggs, almond milk, yogurt and honey. Pour the wet ingredients into the dry ingredients and mix until well combined.. Pour the batter into the prepared loaf pan and bake for 30-35 minutes, or

until a toothpick inserted into the center comes out clean. Allow the bread to cool before slicing and serving.

Sprouted Gluten-Free Buckwheat Bread

Ingredients:

1 cup buckwheat flour

1/2 cup sprouted buckwheat groats

1/4 cup almond flour

1/4 cup tapioca flour

3 tbsp plain yogurt

1 tsp baking soda

1 tbsp lemon juice

1/2 tsp sea salt

2 eggs

1/4 cup coconut oil, melted

1/4 cup honey

Instructions:

Preheat your oven to 350°F and grease a loaf pan. In a large mixing bowl, combine buckwheat flour, sprouted buckwheat groats, almond flour, tapioca flour, baking soda, and sea salt. In a separate bowl, whisk together eggs, melted coconut oil, lemon juice, yogurt and honey. Pour the wet ingredients into the dry ingredients and mix until well combined. Pour the batter into the prepared loaf pan and bake for 40-45 minutes, or until a toothpick inserted into the center comes out clean. Allow the bread to cool before slicing and serving.

Sprouted Gluten-Free Sorghum Bread

Ingredients:

1 cup sorghum flour

1/2 cup sprouted sorghum grains

1/4 cup arrowroot flour

1/4 cup coconut flour

1 tsp baking powder

1/2 tsp sea salt

2 eggs

1/4 cup coconut milk

3 tbsp plain yogurt

2 tbsp maple syrup

Instructions:

Preheat your oven to 350°F and grease a loaf pan. In a large mixing bowl, combine sorghum flour, sprouted sorghum grains, arrowroot flour, coconut flour, baking powder, and sea salt. In a separate bowl, whisk together eggs, coconut milk, yogurt and maple syrup. Pour the wet ingredients into the dry ingredients and mix until well combined. Pour the batter into the prepared loaf pan and bake for 35-40 minutes, or until a toothpick inserted into the center comes out clean. Allow the bread to cool before slicing and serving.

Sprouted Gluten-Free Millet Bread

Ingredients:

1 cup millet flour

1/2 cup sprouted millet seeds

1/4 cup almond flour

1/4 cup oat flour

3 tbsp yogurt

1 tsp baking soda

1/2 tsp sea salt

2 eggs

1/4 cup olive oil

2 tbsp agave nectar

Instructions:

Preheat your oven to 350°F and grease a loaf pan. In a large mixing bowl, combine millet flour, sprouted millet seeds, almond flour, oat flour, baking soda, and sea salt. In a separate bowl, whisk together eggs, olive oil, yogurt and agave nectar. Pour the wet ingredients into the dry ingredients and mix until well combined. Pour the batter into the prepared loaf pan and bake for 30-35 minutes, or

until a toothpick inserted into the center comes out clean. Allow the bread to cool before slicing and serving.

Sprouted Gluten-Free Teff Bread

Ingredients:

1 cup teff flour

1/2 cup sprouted teff grains

1/4 cup arrowroot flour

1/4 cup almond flour

1 tsp baking powder

1/2 tsp sea salt

2 eggs

1/4 cup coconut oil, melted

2 tbsp molasses

Instructions:

Preheat your oven to 350°F and grease a loaf pan. In a large mixing bowl, combine teff flour, sprouted teff grains, arrowroot flour, almond flour, baking powder, and sea salt. In a separate bowl, whisk together eggs, melted coconut oil, and molasses. Pour the wet ingredients into the dry ingredients and mix until well combined. Pour the batter into the prepared loaf pan and bake for 40-45 minutes, or

until a toothpick inserted into the center comes out clean. Allow the bread to cool before slicing and serving.

Rosemary Olive Bread

Ingredients:

2 cups gluten-free all-purpose flour

1 tsp sea salt

 1 tbsp baking powder

1 tsp dried rosemary

1/2 cup sliced black olives

2 eggs

1/4 cup olive oil

1 cup almond milk

Instructions:

Preheat your oven to 350°F (180°C) and grease a loaf pan with olive oil or line it with parchment paper. In a large mixing bowl, combine the gluten-free flour, sea salt, baking powder, and dried rosemary. Add the sliced black olives to the dry ingredients and mix well to ensure the olives are evenly distributed. In a separate bowl, whisk together the eggs, olive oil, and almond milk. Gradually pour the wet ingredients into the dry ingredients, stirring until well combined. The dough should be thick and sticky.

Transfer the dough into the prepared loaf pan, smoothing the top with a spatula. Bake in the preheated oven for 45-50 minutes, or until the bread is golden brown and a toothpick inserted into the center comes out clean. Allow the bread to cool in the pan for 10 minutes before transferring it to a wire rack to cool completely. Slice and serve the rosemary olive gluten-free bread with your favorite spreads or toppings. Enjoy!

Gluten-Free Banana Bread

Ingredients:

1 cup gluten-free oat flour

1 tsp baking soda

1 tbsp apple cider vinegar

1/4 tsp sea salt

3 ripe bananas, mashed

1/4 cup melted coconut oil

1/4 cup maple syrup

1 tsp vanilla extract

2 eggs

Instructions:

Preheat the oven to 350°F (175°C) and grease a loaf pan. In a medium bowl, mix together the gluten-free oat flour, baking soda, and sea salt. In a separate bowl, mix the mashed bananas, coconut oil, maple syrup, vanilla extract, apple cider vinegar and eggs. Combine the wet and dry ingredients until mixed. Pour the batter into the loaf pan and bake for 50-60 minutes, or until a toothpick inserted into the center comes out clean. Let the bread cool before slicing and serving.

Banana Walnut Bread

Ingredients:

2 ripe bananas, mashed

1/3 cup melted butter

3/4 cup sugar

1 egg, beaten

1 tsp vanilla extract

1 tsp baking soda

Pinch of sea salt

 1 tbsp lemon juice

1 1/2 cups gluten free oat flour

1/2 cup chopped walnuts

Instructions:

Preheat the oven to 350°F (175°C) and grease a loaf pan. In a large bowl, mix together the mashed bananas, melted butter, sugar, egg, lemon juice and vanilla extract. Add the baking soda, sea salt, and oat flour, and mix until just combined. Fold in the chopped walnuts.

Pour the batter into the loaf pan and bake for 60-70 minutes, or until a toothpick inserted into the center comes out clean. Let the bread cool before slicing and serving.

Sweet Potato Bread

Ingredients:

1 cup mashed sweet potato

1/2 cup sugar

1/4 cup melted coconut oil

1/4 cup almond milk

1 tsp vanilla extract

1 1/4 cups gluten-free oat flour

1 tsp baking powder

1/2 tsp baking soda

1/2 tsp cinnamon

1/4 tsp sea salt

Instructions:

Preheat the oven to 350°F (175°C) and grease a loaf pan. In a large bowl, mix together the mashed sweet potato, sugar, coconut oil, almond milk, and vanilla extract. In a separate bowl, whisk together the gluten-free oat flour, baking powder, baking soda, cinnamon, and sea salt. Combine the wet and dry ingredients until mixed well. Pour the batter into the loaf pan and bake for 45-50 minutes, or until a toothpick inserted into the center comes out clean.

Gluten Free Chickpea Bread

Ingredients:

2 cups chickpea flour

1 cup water

1/4 cup olive oil

1 tsp sea salt

1 tsp baking powder

Instructions:

Preheat the oven to 350°F (180°C) and grease a loaf pan. In a mixing bowl, combine the chickpea flour, water, olive oil, sea salt, and baking powder. Whisk well until a smooth batter forms. Pour the batter into the greased loaf pan and smooth the top with a spatula. Bake in the preheated oven for 30-35 minutes, or until a toothpick inserted into the enter comes out clean. Let the bread cool in the pan for 10 minutes before transferring it to a wire rack to cool completely.

Buckwheat Bread

Ingredients:

2 cups buckwheat flour

3 tablespoon yogurt

1/4 cup ground flax meal

1 tsp sea salt

1 tsp baking powder

1/4 cup olive oil

1 cup water

Instructions:

Preheat the oven to 350°F (180°C) and grease a loaf pan. In a mixing bowl, combine the buckwheat flour, ground flax meal, sea salt, and baking powder. Mix well. Add the yogurt, olive oil and water to the dry ingredients and mix until a smooth batter forms. Pour the batter into the greased loaf pan and smooth the top with a spatula. Bake in the preheated oven for 40-45 minutes, or until a toothpick inserted into the center comes out clean. Let the bread cool in the pan for 10 minutes before transferring it to a wire rack to cool completely.

Flax Seed Bread

Ingredients:

2 cups almond flour

1/2 cup ground flax seeds

1/4 cup coconut flour

1 tsp baking soda

3 tbsp plain yogurt

1 tsp sea salt

4 eggs

1/4 cup olive oil

1/4 cup water

Instructions:

Preheat the oven to 350°F (180°C) and grease a loaf pan. In a mixing bowl, combine the almond flour, ground flax seeds, coconut flour, baking soda, and sea salt. Mix well. In a separate bowl, whisk together the eggs, olive oil, yogurt and water. Pour the wet ingredients into the dry ingredients and mix until well combined. Pour the batter into the greased loaf pan and smooth the top with a spatula. Bake in the preheated oven for 45-50 minutes, or until a toothpick inserted into the center comes out clean. Let the bread cool in the pan for 10 minutes before transferring it to a wire rack to cool completely.

Garlic Bread

Ingredients:

1 loaf of gluten free bread (store-bought or homemade)

1/2 cup butter or margarine

3 cloves garlic, minced

1/4 cup fresh parsley, chopped

Salt and pepper, to taste

Instructions:

Preheat the oven to 350°F (180°C). In a small saucepan, melt the butter or margarine over low heat. Add the minced garlic and cook for 1-2 minutes, until fragrant. Stir in the chopped parsley, salt, and pepper. Cut the loaf of gluten free bread into thick slices and place on a baking sheet. Brush the garlic butter mixture onto each bread slice. Bake in the preheated oven for 3-5minutes, or until the bread is toasted and the garlic butter is melted. Serve warm and enjoy!

Zucchini Bread

Ingredients:

2 cups grated zucchini

3/4 cup almond flour

1/4 cup coconut flour

1/4 cup ground flax meal

3 tbsp Greek yogurt

1 tsp baking powder

1 tsp baking soda

1 tsp cinnamon

1/4 tsp sea salt

3 eggs

1/4 cup maple syrup

1/4 cup coconut oil, melted

1 tsp vanilla extract

Instructions:

Preheat the oven to 350°F (180°C) and grease a loaf pan. In a mixing bowl, combine the grated zucchini, almond flour, coconut flour, ground flax meal, baking powder, baking soda, cinnamon, and sea salt. Mix well. In a separate bowl, whisk together the eggs, maple syrup, yogurt melted coconut oil, and vanilla extract. Pour the wet ingredients into the dry ingredients and mix until well combined.

92

Pour the batter into the greased loaf pan and smooth the top with a spatula. Bake in the preheated oven for 50-55 minutes, or until a toothpick inserted into the center comes out clean. Let the bread cool in the pan for 10 minutes before transferring it to a wire rack to cool completely.

Pumpkin Bread

Ingredients:

1 cup pumpkin puree

2 eggs

1/4 cup coconut oil, melted

1/4 cup maple syrup

1 tsp vanilla extract

1 1/2 cups oat flour

1/4 cup almond flour

1 tsp baking powder

1 tsp cinnamon

1/2 tsp nutmeg

1/4 tsp cloves

1/4 tsp sea salt

Instructions:

Preheat the oven to 350°F (180°C) and grease a loaf pan. In a mixing bowl, combine the pumpkin puree, eggs, melted coconut oil, maple syrup, and vanilla extract. Mix well. Add the almond flour, oat flour, baking powder, cinnamon, nutmeg, cloves, and sea salt to the wet ingredients. Mix until well combined. Pour the batter into the greased loaf pan and smooth the top with a spatula.

Bake in the preheated oven for 50-55 minutes, or until a toothpick inserted into the center comes out clean. Let the bread cool in the pan for 10 minutes before transferring it to a wire rack to cool completely.

ABOUT THE AUTHOR

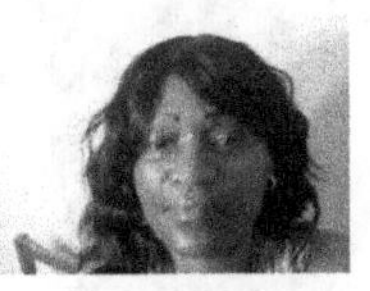

Pansy Worthy a talented Mom behind "Bread Without Gluten: Easy And Delicious Recipes for a Gluten-Free Lifestyle"! She is a passionate home baker who was inspired to create this cookbook after her son was diagnosed with digestive disorder and discovering the limited options available for gluten free bread.

Pansy's journey to creating delicious gluten-free bread recipes started out of necessity, but it quickly evolved into a passion project. She spent countless hours in her kitchen experimenting with different free flours rising agents and techniques to develop recipes that were not only safe for those with digestive issues, but also tasted just as good as traditional bread.

With a background in health and nutrition and a love for baking, Pansy was able to bring a unique perspective to gluten free bread making. She understands the importance of using wholesome, nutritious ingredients that not only taste great, but also support overall health and well-being.

 Pansy's cookbook is a testament to her dedication to helping others with gluten sensitivities enjoy delicious bread without sacrificing taste or texture. Her recipes are easy to follow, with clear instructions for both beginners and experienced bakers.

BOOKS BY THE AUTHOR

Gut Health and Diseases: A Guide to Gut Healing and Digestive Disorders

Gut health is essential for overall well-being, as the gut plays a crucial role indigestion, immune function, and mental health. In this comprehensive guide, readers will learn everything they need to know about maintaining a healthy gut and preventing diseases arising from gut imbalances.

From the importance of gut bacteria to the connection between gut health and chronic diseases like obesity, diabetes, mental illness, and autoimmune disorders, this book covers it all.

Juicing For The Special Needs Child & Family

In Juicing For The Special Needs Child & Family" is not just a recipe book; it's a life-enhancing resource that equips parents and caregivers with helpful tools to navigate the particular dietary needs of their special needs child. From understanding juicing basics and its benefits to identifying specific juice recipes for specific health issues with nutrients that can support cognitive function and overall well-being, this book covers it all.

GLUTEN FREE & SUGAR FREE BAKING: FOR THE SPECIAL NEEDS CHILD & FAMILY

Gluten-Free & Sugar-Free Baking For The Special Need Child & Family cookbook was created by a mom with a son diagnosed with autism and severe mental disabilities around the age of 6. This cookbook is focused on preparing meals for the entire family instead of one individual. I know firsthand the pressure of buying many different ingredients and preparing multiple meals for different members of the family. It is stressful, expensive, time-consuming, and creates a burden on the caregiver.

The book features all recipes that you can bake. Over 80 recipes include bread, cake, muffin, cookie, cupcakes, brownies, pizza, wraps, donuts, garlic knots, rolls, bagels, and more. They are fun and easy to make even a child can make them.